Masks & Scrubs

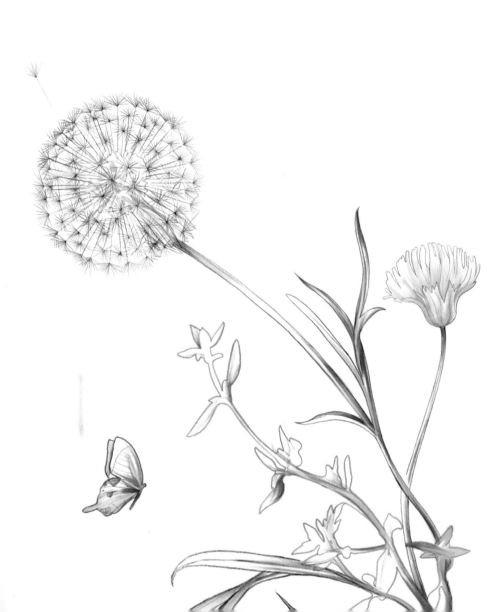

WHOLE BEAUTY

Masks & Scrubs

Natural Beauty Recipes for Ultimate Self-Care

SHIVA ROSE

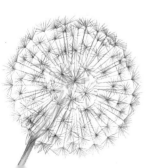

ARTISAN I NEW YORK

CONTENTS

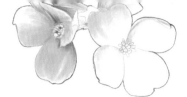

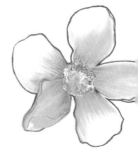

Introduction:
My Whole Beauty Practices

I spend hours in our garden, gathering pansies,
roses, cherry blossoms, and all the other vivid,
scented plants that catch my eye. I collect the
petals in a small copper bowl, add a little water
from the pond, and with a pestle, mash them
until they form a fragrant and vibrant paste.

I take my seat at the edge of the pond and dangle my
feet in, piquing the curiosity of the goldfish, sending
them swimming to ripple the lily pads across the
surface. I take my flower paste and rub it on my
face, breathing in the aroma of the flowers. This
is Iran, this is the beginning, but if I close my eyes
now, many years and thousands of miles away in Los
Angeles, I am there again. I can still feel the wind on
my cheeks and the tickle of fish nibbling at my toes
and hear birds singing as they dance by overhead.

I was young enough that I didn't think of these
pondside rituals as beautifying or acts of self-care.
I just saw them as a way to bring myself even closer
to the natural world, reveling in the way the yellows,
reds, and purples looked before my eyes and how
soft the petals felt as I crushed them with my hands.

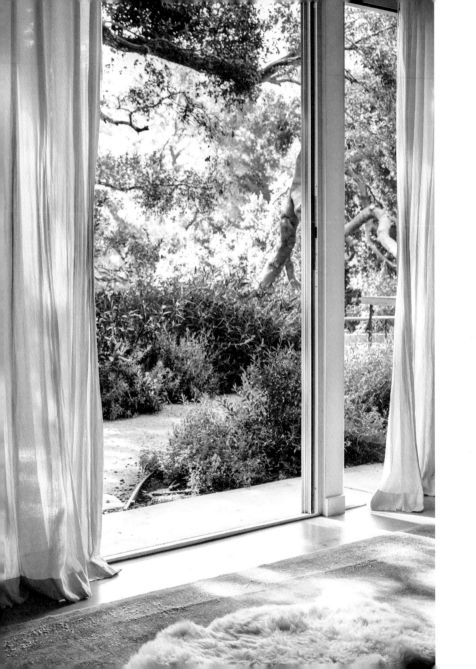

It was a pure moment of creation that amplified my senses and gave me a small gift of beauty to carry with me even when I was called away from the garden.

Approaching beauty with reverence and ritual can help awaken your feminine fire and stoke the flames of vibrancy and passion. Creating rituals to acknowledge and induce pleasure is a form of religion, a way to care as much for the soul as for the skin and it is the simplest and biggest way you can honor yourself and enhance your well-being. The rituals you create will transform self-care from a chore into an act of love.

Beauty Recipes

You make your own food because you care about what you put into your body, so why wouldn't you make what you put *on* your body with equal reverence and care? While conventional products may work for a short amount of time, many of them will cause harm in the long run, and I truly believe that beauty and self-care are cumulative. There is no quick fix.

Taking the time to make your own products is a way of pausing the frenetic pace of modern life. It is an act of creation that provides an experience far more personal and sensual than just unscrewing the lid of a jar. Creativity has no judgment, and it can morph into anything. You connect with the ingredients through sight, touch, smell, and taste, and as you become the alchemist of your own beauty, the flow takes over. You experiment with scents and textures, adding new elements that speak to what you need. When you are done, you hold in your hands something that will not just beautify your skin or hair but also transform your whole being.

The recipes in this book are here as a way for you to sensually indulge your skin and hair, using ingredients that you often have on hand. There is no right way to use these recipes. Doing so is a personal experience. And at the heart of these recipes and beauty rituals is allowing our intuition the space to breathe and blossom and lead us to what our bodies need.

Some of the recipes here incorporate Ayurvedic principles. Ayurveda is an Indian healing modality that is thousands of years old. Its focus is on preventing illness by constantly cleansing and detoxifying the body. In Ayurveda, inner and outer beauty are intimately related. I truly believe that beautifying ourselves holistically is an integral part of self-care, health, and healing. Beauty that does not penetrate beyond the first, physical layer will fade, but beauty that comes from being nourished and balanced spiritually, emotionally, and physically radiates from the eyes, hair, and every pore.

Generally, the recipes are very safe, but use caution if you have allergies or sensitive skin. If there is anything that you think you might be allergic to or that might cause harm, it is a good idea to test it on the inside of your arm. You can apply the oil, essential oil, or ingredient to the skin (wash it off if it is a mask component) and wait twenty-four hours to see if any irritation develops.

Make the most of this step on your wellness journey by creating some time for you; get messy and enjoy.

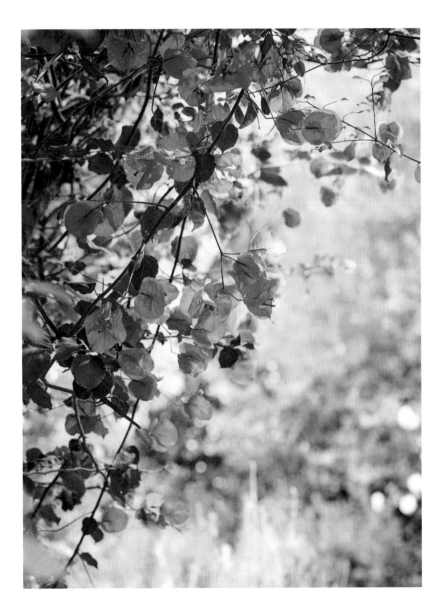

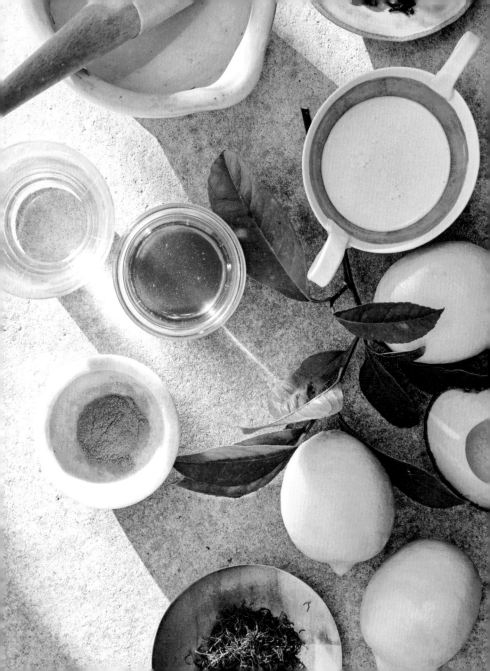

My Pantry Is My Beauty Counter

Being able to turn to the kitchen when you need something for your skin or hair is inexpensive and convenient, and since the ingredients are natural and edible, they can be used without risk of damage or irritation (see page 10). Each self-care product is a story, and the ingredients are the characters. The magic is in how they come together, to complement and contrast with one another. There is no right or wrong way to mix natural ingredients. You can add or subtract based on what your skin or hair needs at the moment, and to suit your preference.

Following are the items you'll always find in my pantry.

Aloe

Most of us know aloe from using it to soothe a sunburn, and its cooling effects come from hormones that help heal wounds and calm inflammation. You can also drink aloe juice from time to time to deliver these same effects to your entire body.

Amla Fruit

This beautiful Indian fruit ripens on the
tree and bursts open in autumn. It is full of
antioxidants and also provides many nutrients.
It can help skin, hair, and hormonal balance,
and it will continue to give and give.

Apple Cider Vinegar

Apple cider vinegar has been used in beauty
rituals since ancient Roman times, and the
empress of Hungary was said to have had
beautiful skin from applying it to her face as a
toner. It is naturally antiseptic and antibacterial,
which makes it great for calming acne, and
it helps to balance the pH of the skin.

Avocados

Avocados are full of good fats and moisture for your
hair and skin, and your body will rejoice in soaking
them up, inside and out. The avocado is such a
dignified fruit with its beautiful emerald-green flesh
that delivers a big caress of lusciousness to your skin.

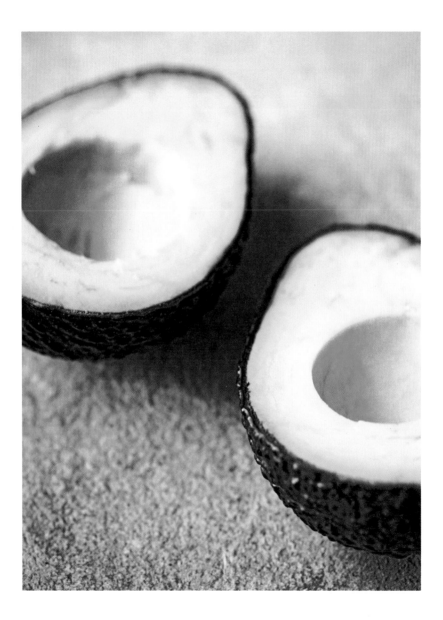

Bananas

Bananas are full of potassium, which helps to strengthen hair, repairing damage and preventing breakage. They are also full of powerful antioxidants like vitamins A, C, and E and zinc, which can prevent aging and nourish the skin.

Bhringaraj

Bhringaraj symbolizes reverence for the sacred masculine. It promotes hair growth and luster and also calms the nervous system.

Egg Yolks

Egg yolks are rich in sulfur content, which helps in relieving dandruff symptoms and in maintaining a healthy scalp. Eggs are a wonderful source of protein and lecithin, both of which aid in moisturizing and strengthening hair. Lecithin acts as a natural emulsifier, which means that it binds together the ingredients of a homemade hair mask and converts them into a homogenous mixture.

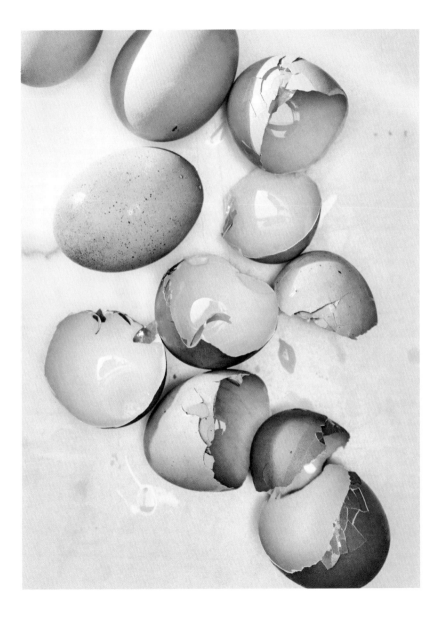

Green Tea

Green tea is rich in powerful antioxidants,
and applied topically, it helps to flush toxins
from the skin and reduce inflammation.

Honey

In ancient Greek myths, honey was called ambrosia,
the food of the gods. The humble bees who work
so hard to create this elixir of life are always
feeding us. Honey is sweet and dewy, a balm for
our skin, our soul, and the planet. It's simply divine,
and also antibacterial and super moisturizing, so
it can help calm acne and give your skin a glow.
Use raw honey, as processed honey has been
stripped of its beneficial probiotics and enzymes.

Lemons

I love to drive through Ojai and smell the fresh
neroli and lemon blossoms scenting the air.
Bright and energetic, lemons remind me of the
sun, and just a whiff of them can create that
happy energy in your mind. Lemons can also
serve as an excellent toner for your skin.

Nutmeg

Nutmeg is known in Ayurveda for its antiseptic and antiviral properties, which make it great for helping to heal acne and reduce scarring.

Papaya

Called "fruit of the angels" by Christopher Columbus, papaya is full of papain enzymes, which help clear away dead cells as well as feed your skin with vitamins A, C, and E.

Pearl Powder

Pearl powder reminds me of moon dust, and yet it comes from seashells in the ocean. It feeds us with minerals that we are lacking so that we can shine like iridescent moon pearls.

Pineapple

Pineapple is one of many tropical fruits that are full of antioxidants and exfoliating enzymes to make you glow.

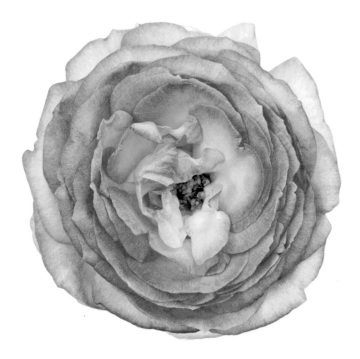

Raw Milk

Unlike pasteurized milk, raw milk still contains
a lot of the good bacteria and enzymes that will
feed your skin. Now more and more dairies are
producing raw milk, and there are food co-ops
that sell it. Finding it might take a bit of research,
but it will be well worth it! If you can't find raw
milk, make sure you are using organic milk that
has not been treated with any hormones.

Roses

Roses are the queen of all flowers, with a
higher measure of chi than any other. Mother
Mary is represented by the rose, the most
divine flower of all. It is wonderful for the skin,
the heart, the soul, and the spirit. Rose oil,
crushed rose petals, and rose hip oil are all anti-
aging, moisturizing, and anti-inflammatory.

Royal Jelly

As a beekeeper, I have such a reverence for the
bees. Hair can become brittle from the water and
the air, and rubbing just a little bit of royal jelly—a
secretion of worker bees that feeds the larvae
and is full of amino acids and protein—through
the strands of your hair or the roots at the scalp

and allowing those precious nutrients to soak in can give you luscious locks. Rich in protein; vitamins B_1, B_2, and B_6; biotin; and folic acid, royal jelly is wonderful for rejuvenating the scalp and helping to prevent prematurely gray hair.

Saffron

O saffron, you represent the nights of Persia. You smell like summer and you shine like the bright sun. Grains of white rice become a celebration when touched by your golden hue. You illuminate the face and open the heart to a feeling of endless possibility. Saffron is a magical ingredient that does wonders for clarifying the skin and evening out its tone. Just smelling a few silken red strands will awaken you to the powers of this magical ingredient.

Sandalwood Powder

Not only does sandalwood have a beautiful, uplifting scent, but it also reduces pigmentation and scarring and helps to heal blemishes.

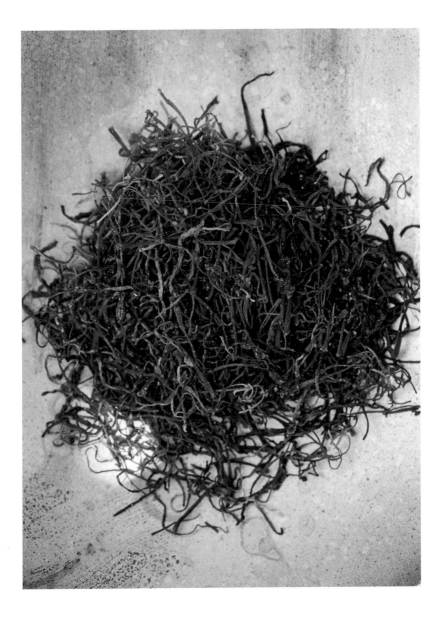

Shatavari

Shatavari is a wonder herb from India that is especially good for women. It makes your hair shine and your skin glow, and it calms your hormones.

Shikakai

Shikakai is an Ayurvedic herb that is often used to cleanse the hair because of its astringent, anti-dandruff properties. It is also rich in vitamins A, C, and K, which aid in nourishing the hair.

Turmeric

Turmeric is like powdered gold and sunshine. When used on the skin or taken internally, it can create optimal health and vibrancy and help heal and prevent inflammation. The wealth of the earth is given to us through turmeric.

Water

Having access to clean water should be so simple. Sadly, it is not. For those of us who are fortunate enough to live in a place where the tap water is potable, we know it is still very rarely healthy and has often been treated with chemicals such as chlorine and fluoride. When water is bottled in plastic, chemicals can leach from the packaging into the water, leading to liver and kidney stagnation and toxic buildup. It's preferable to have a water filtration system installed in your home, buy water in glass bottles, or get water directly from a spring. Mountain Valley and Castle Rock are two brands that I like, and FindASpring.com can help you locate spring water in your area.

Yogurt

Creamy yogurt is like a sweet, cooling embrace on a hot summer day. It is alive, full of beneficial enzymes and probiotics, and is a superfood for your skin. Plain yogurt contains zinc, which is anti-inflammatory and promotes cell reproduction; lactic acid, which is mildly exfoliating and great for wrinkles; calcium, which is an antioxidant and facilitates skin renewal; and B vitamins, which help keep skin glowing. You can mix yogurt with other ingredients to make a mask, or use it solo as a moisturizing treat for skin and hair.

A note on using ingredients produced by animals: It is always important to give gratitude—to the industrious bees that created the honey, to the chickens that laid the eggs. I like to pour a little of their gift on the earth as a reminder to be grateful.

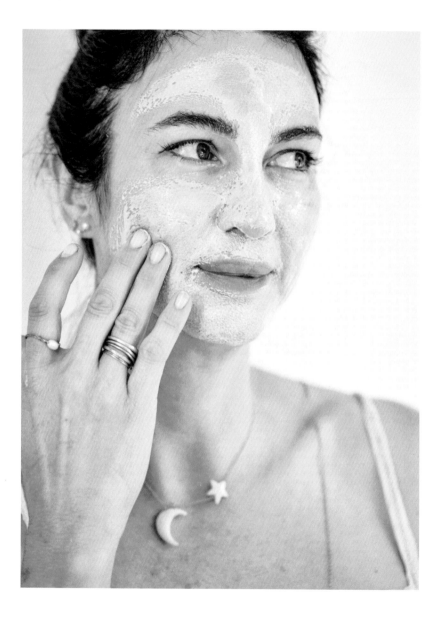

Facial Treatments

We need to treat our facial skin with even more tenderness and grace than we do the skin on the rest of our body. It is even more susceptible to wrinkles and discoloration, and the skin around the eyes can be especially fragile. Because our face is what we see when we look in the mirror, and it is where we house many of our most powerful characteristics, I feel like we are honoring our entire being when we show devotion to this one part of our body. I love getting facial treatments from professional aestheticians, but I find these do-it-yourself facial treatments to be just as healing. And feeling the ingredients mush between your fingers and smelling the spices as you stir will activate your spirit more than anything you could buy at the store. I find it wonderfully satisfying to create a sensual, beautifying experience, full of self-love, from ingredients I already have in my kitchen.

The treatments on the following pages are gentle enough that they can be used on all skin types, but each one notes which type of skin it will be most beneficial for. All of the recipes make one treatment, so feel free to double or triple them as needed to beautify with friends.

Plumping Goddess
Nectar Mask

This mask is rich, creamy, and sensuous, full of beneficial fats that can help imbue parched skin with moisture. Caring for your skin shouldn't be a clinical process, and making this mask should be a very visceral experience. Really smoosh it around and feel it with your fingers as you're mixing it.

For
Dry and mature skin types

Recommended Use
Once a week, to feed your skin and being

¼ cup avocado
¼ cup mashed banana
¼ cup raw honey
¼ cup plain yogurt

Using your fingers, mix the avocado, banana, honey, and yogurt in a bowl until they are well combined (the mixture should be a pale green). Wash your face and pat it dry, then slowly and lovingly apply the mixture. (Any leftover mask can be used on your hair and the rest of your body.) Leave on for 20 minutes, then rinse off with cool water.

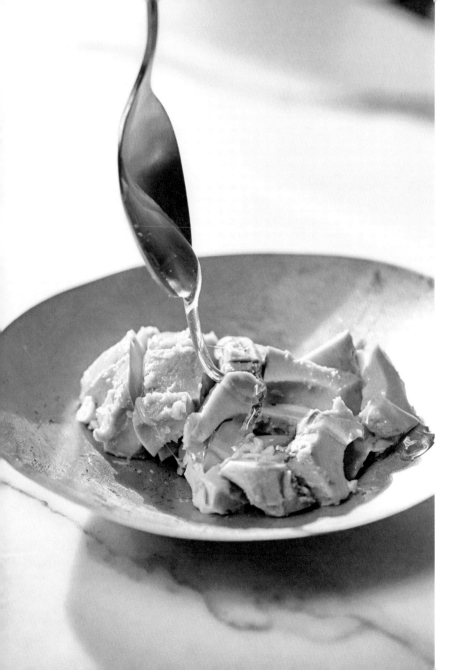

Exfoliating Luscious Island Mask

Pineapples, papayas, mangoes, coconuts, and lychees don't last long in our house, but whatever we don't eat, I use to make masks. The acids in these tropical fruits are gentle exfoliators, and bromelain, an enzyme that's derived from pineapples, is really good for inflammation.

For

All skin types, though use caution if your skin is sensitive. Natural alpha hydroxy acids and enzymes are safer than chemicals, but they can still cause irritation.

Recommended Use

Once a month to leave your skin with a radiant glow

¼ cup papaya or pineapple (pineapple is stronger, but papaya seeds can also be added for extra exfoliation)
¼ cup plain yogurt

Mix the fruit and yogurt together in a bowl with a wooden spoon, using the back of the spoon to mash the fruit. It's okay if there are some chunks. Wash your face and pat it dry, then spread the mask on with your fingers. Leave on for 15 minutes, then rinse off with warm water.

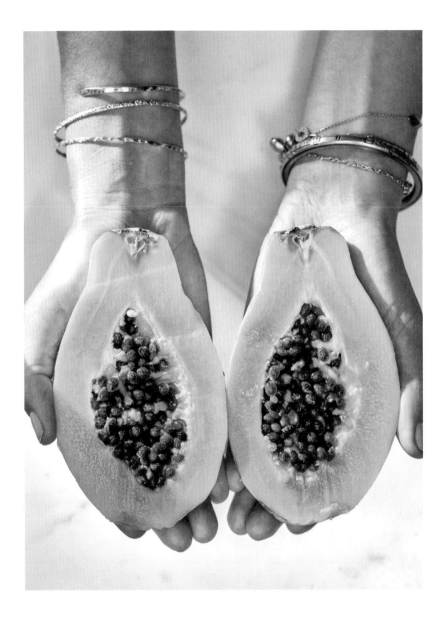

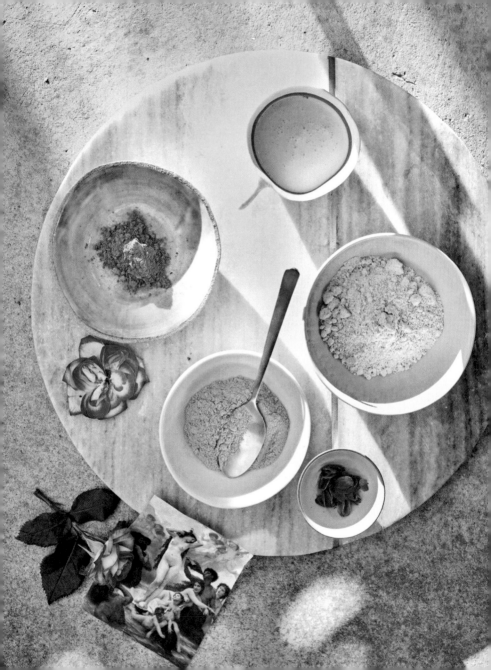

Venus Beauty Mask

Women are ruled by Venus, who is all about love, compassion, and prosperity. In Persian and Ayurvedic teachings, sandalwood opens your third eye chakra (located in the center of your forehead) and rose opens your heart, and together, they uplift your spirits. Astringent sandalwood cools with antibacterial properties that help prevent acne, while rose petals deliver anti-aging moisture. I love how beautiful and indulgent this mask feels as it balances skin and makes it absolutely glow.

For
Normal to dry skin types

Recommended Use
Twice a month or as needed to moisturize

5 tablespoons oat flour
3 tablespoons milk, preferably raw (see page 21)
1 teaspoon sandalwood powder
A small handful of crushed dried rose petals, plus
    1 teaspoon ground

Mix the oat flour with the milk in a bowl and stir until it forms a paste. Sprinkle in the sandalwood powder and rose petals. Stir until you achieve a smooth consistency. Wash your face and pat it dry, then apply the mask using upward strokes. Leave on for 20 minutes, then rinse off with warm water.

Cooling Milk &
Spice Mask

Breakouts are eruptions usually caused by too much Pitta—fire energy—in the body. We have to learn how to harness the passion and fire and put it to work for us. Otherwise, we just swallow that fire, which creates hormonal issues that manifest as acne or cysts. This mask treats acne by soothing and calming the skin to leave it smooth and supple. The medicinal qualities of nutmeg help to rejuvenate the skin and also treat anxiety and digestive issues in the body. Whole milk is full of nourishing fats that help moisturize, and when these two ingredients are mixed together, your skin will want to drink up the combination. (In fact, it is good enough that you could drink it!)

For

Oily and acne-prone skin types

Recommended Use

Two or three times a month, if you have a lot of breakouts

Continued

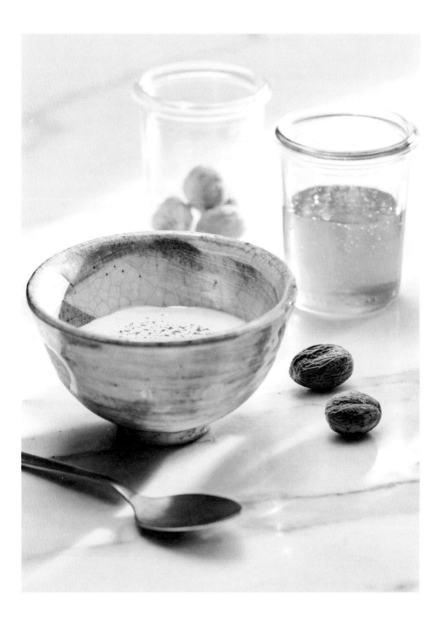

2 or 3 whole nutmeg pods, or 1 tablespoon
    ground nutmeg
1 tablespoon whole milk, preferably raw (see page 19),
    plus more as needed
1 teaspoon raw honey (optional; use only if you have
    exceptionally oily skin)

Grind the whole nutmeg in a coffee grinder and
transfer to a bowl. Add the milk and the honey, if
using, and stir until combined to form a paste. You
can add water instead of more milk to get the right
consistency. Wash your face and pat it dry, then
apply the mask all over or just to problem areas. You
may get some tingling, but that means the mask is
being activated. Leave on for 15 to 20 minutes, then
rinse off with cool water.

Golden Sun Mask

This mask really makes you radiant, like the sun. It combines three of my favorite ingredients— yogurt, honey, and saffron—and it's a mix of Persian and Ayurvedic traditions. The unusual flavor and beautiful golden red color of saffron come from the crocus flower, and it is said that it takes 4,500 crocus flowers to make one ounce of saffron. Ayurvedic practices call on saffron for its incredible healing properties in everything from reducing stress and depression to soothing menstrual cramps and even helping with male fertility issues. It also helps alleviate skin discoloration, dullness, and acne. This mask will brighten your skin for a special occasion, birthday, holiday, or romantic date.

For
Normal to dry skin types

Recommended Use
As needed for special occasions

½ cup plain yogurt (preferably goat's or sheep's milk)
3 tablespoons raw honey
1 tablespoon saffron threads

Combine the yogurt, honey, and saffron in a bowl and stir until the mixture is a pale golden hue. Wash your face and pat it dry, then brush the mask onto your

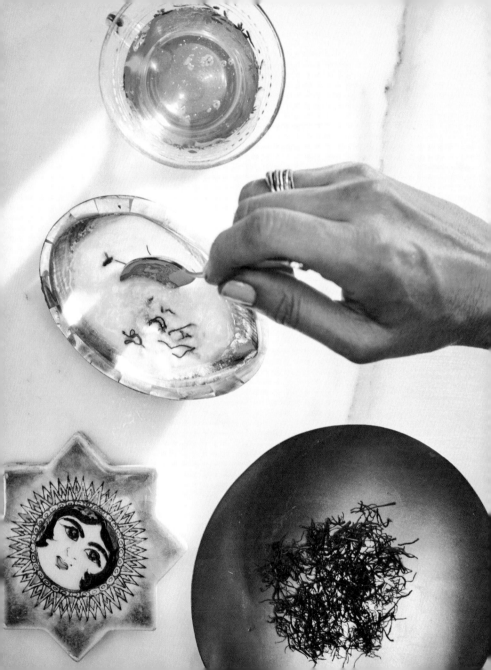

skin. Leave on for 15 to 20 minutes, then rinse off
with lukewarm water.

Exfoliating Version

By hand, squeeze a few drops of lemon juice into
the mixture and add 1 teaspoon of organic sugar.
(I like to use coconut sugar.) Mix well and let sit for
10 minutes before applying. Pat on, using circular,
upward motions. Leave on for 15 to 20 minutes, then
rinse off with lukewarm water. Lemon will make the
mask more lightening, and sugar helps to exfoliate.

Chaga Power Mask

Chaga is called "the king of medicinal mushrooms." Though it's not much to look at, chaga has more antioxidants than pomegranates and blueberries, which makes this mask like a superfood for your skin. It can help fight everything from premature aging and sun damage to broken capillaries and hyperpigmentation. You can get chaga at most health food stores, and it usually comes in raw form (chunks) or powder.

For
Mature or sun-damaged skin

Recommended Use
Once or twice a month

1 tablespoon chaga chunks, or
   2 tablespoons chaga powder
2 tablespoons raw honey
2 tablespoons coconut oil

If using chaga chunks, place 1 cup water in a saucepan, drop in the chaga, and bring to a boil. Reduce the heat and let simmer for at least an hour, or until the water has condensed slightly and turns a deep brown.

If using chaga powder, stir it into 1 cup boiling water, then allow to cool.

Mix the cooled chaga "tea" with the honey and coconut oil in a bowl. Wash your face and pat it dry, then apply the mask. Leave on for 15 minutes, then rinse off with lukewarm water.

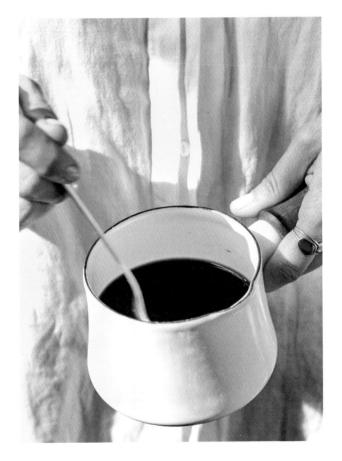

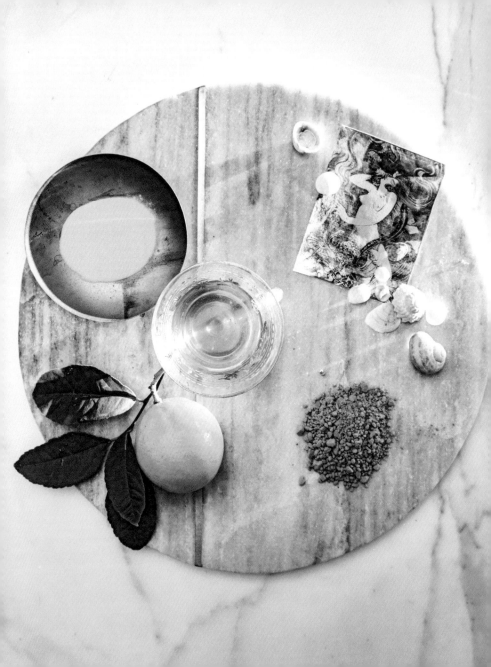

Calming Mineral Mermaid Mask

This mask leaves the skin smooth and hydrated. Plus, it is satisfying and fun to peel off! Agar-agar is derived from seaweed and is full of iron, magnesium, copper, and calcium, all of which make it anti-inflammatory. The honey is also antibacterial.

For
Oily skin

Recommended Use
Once or twice a month, or as needed to calm breakouts

1 cup boiled green tea (use 2 tea bags)
1 tablespoon raw honey
1 tablespoon lemon juice
2 tablespoons agar-agar

Mix together the green tea, honey, lemon juice, and agar-agar in a saucepan and bring to a boil for 2 minutes. Remove from the heat and let sit until it becomes a thick paste. Wash your face and pat it dry, then apply the paste and let it dry. (Any leftover mask can be used on your neck, hands, and feet.) When it has dried, it will have a rubbery texture and you can peel it right off. Use a washcloth and warm water to remove any mask left on your skin.

Blissful Beetroot Lip Balm

When you have glowing, dewy skin, you do not need much makeup—just a reddish-pink lip tint and a light coat of mascara will do.

2 tablespoons beeswax
2 tablespoons cocoa butter
2 tablespoons coconut oil
2 tablespoons beet juice or pureed beet

Small glass container or metal tin with lid

In a small saucepan, melt the beeswax, cocoa butter, and coconut oil over low heat until liquefied. Remove from the heat and whisk in the beet juice or puree. Put the mixture in a blender and blend on high for 30 seconds to emulsify. Transfer the mixture to the container and refrigerate until solid. The lip balm can be kept at room temperature away from direct heat or sunlight for 3 to 4 months or stored in the refrigerator for up to a year.

Tip: This lip balm will melt easily, so be careful about leaving it in your purse on a hot summer day.

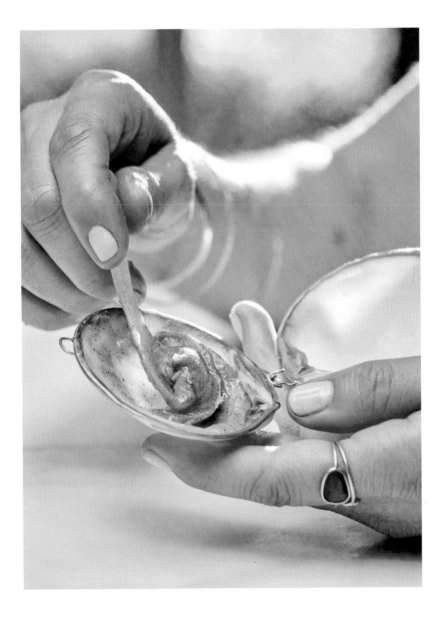

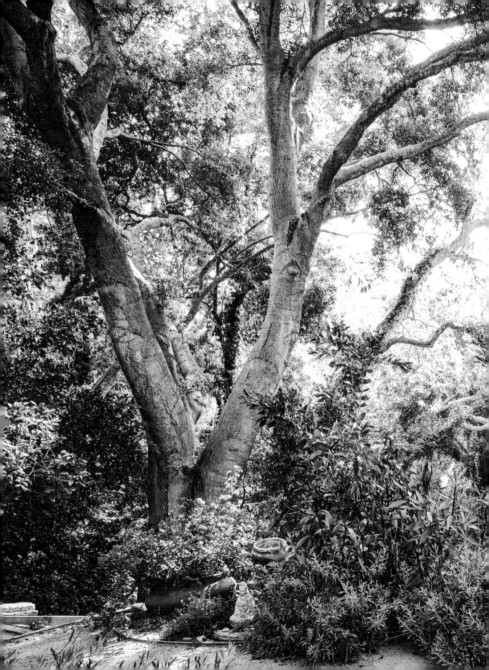

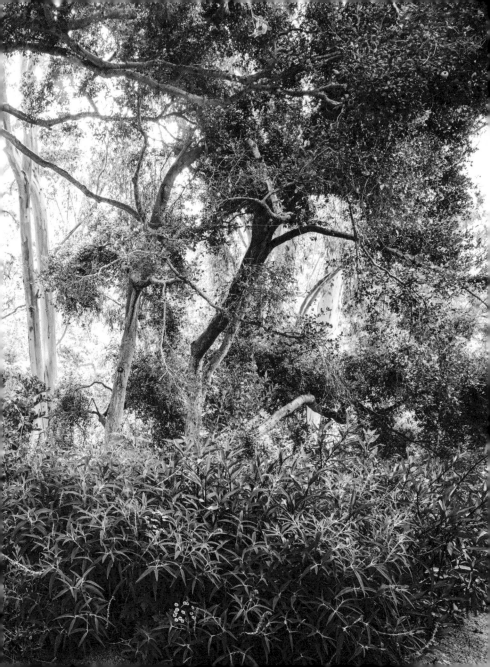

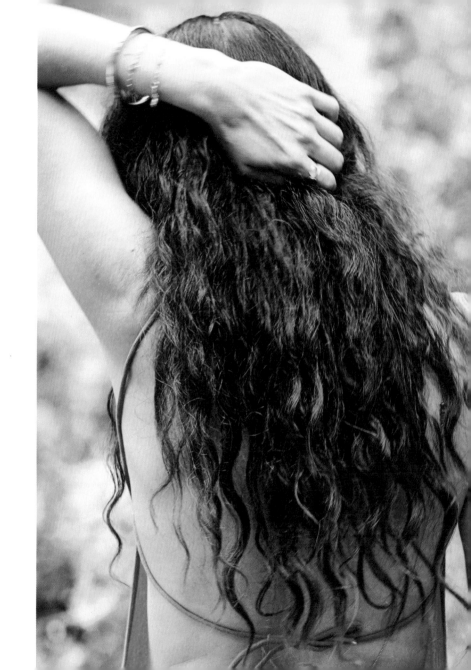

Hair Care

Legend has it that during the Vietnam War, the CIA recruited Native Americans because they were known for their remarkable ability to track animals in even the densest vegetation.

However, once the trackers got to Vietnam, they weren't able to do their work at all. They had lost all of their ability. Why? Because the government had forced them to cut their hair, and with their hair went their power.

I do believe that our hair is connected to our intuition. Our hair is both our antennae and our tail, and a strong communicator. From the Kundalini perspective, the hair is a vibrant source of creative life force that helps to funnel powerful sun energy into the frontal lobes of the brain. Your hair's health, much like your skin's, can alert you to changes in your overall health—specifically hormonal imbalances, thyroid issues, and toxicity buildup—before symptoms are manifested elsewhere in your body.

From goddesses to queens, women have always used their hair to express themselves and their intentions. Whether it's Jean Seberg's pixie cut, Goddess Lalita's thick, dark locks scented with champaca flowers, or Cleopatra's blunt-cut bangs, hair is a source of feminine power, and keeping yours healthy and lustrous will also help your aura shine. Use these treatments to deep-condition your hair before shampooing and conditioning as you normally do.

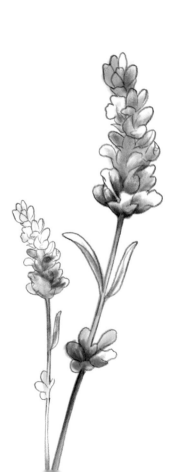

Lustrous Lakshmi Mask

Named for the Hindu goddess of Fortune and prosperity, this mask adds some love to your locks as it conditions, stops dandruff, and makes your hair grow longer, stronger, and faster. It also helps to balance your three doshas, or life-giving forces: Vata, Pitta, and Kapha. According to Ayurveda, when the three doshas are perfectly aligned and balanced, you are considered healthy. Fenugreek seeds are an Indian spice known for their sweet smell and helpfulness in treating hair loss and baldness. Shikakai powder comes from a common Asian shrub and is high in antioxidants like vitamins A, C, and K. It helps to balance the pH of the hair and make it shiny. Amla fruit has three times more vitamin C than an orange. It nourishes hair from the scalp to the ends. If you are having trouble finding these ingredients in your area, you can order them from Banyan Botanicals or Dual Spices (see Resources).

For
All hair types

Recommended Use
Once a month

Continued

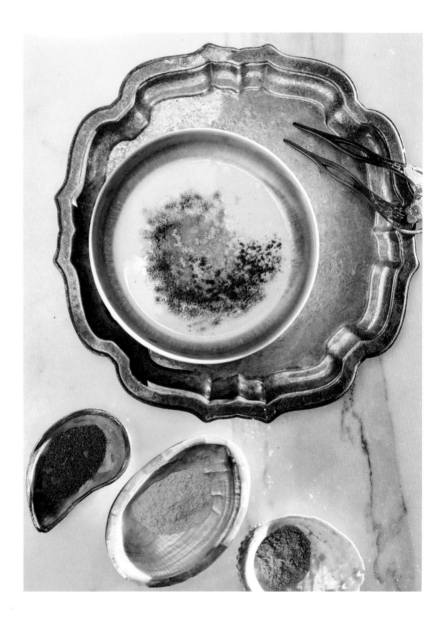

1 tablespoon fenugreek powder

1 tablespoon shikakai powder

2 tablespoons amla fruit powder

2 tablespoons plain yogurt

In a bowl, combine the three powders and add enough water to form a paste (5 or 6 tablespoons should be enough, but add as much as you need to attain the desired consistency). Let the paste sit for a few hours. Stir in the yogurt and let the mixture sit for an hour. Apply to your hair and scalp. Leave on for an hour, then lightly shampoo.

Apple Cider Vinegar Rinse

You'll be amazed at how soft and shiny your hair can be when you rinse it with apple cider vinegar, which acts as a detoxifier. The acidity of apple cider vinegar helps to balance the pH of your hair, and it also strips off the residue left by traditional hair products, leaving the hair unbelievably silky. It has zero harmful chemicals and a price tag far lower than anything you could buy at a salon.

For

All hair types

Recommended Use

Once a month, as a nice reset for the hair

1 tablespoon apple cider vinegar (I love Bragg and
     Fire Cider)
8 ounces water
A few drops of an essential oil, such as rosemary or
     lavender, to stimulate the scalp and help mask the
     pungent scent of the vinegar

Glass jar, cup, or spray bottle

Combine the vinegar, water, and essential oil in the jar, cup, or spray bottle and stir or shake to mix well. Pour over or spray through clean, wet hair. Leave it on for 1 to 2 minutes, then really rinse it out. If you like, apply a traditional conditioner on your ends afterward.

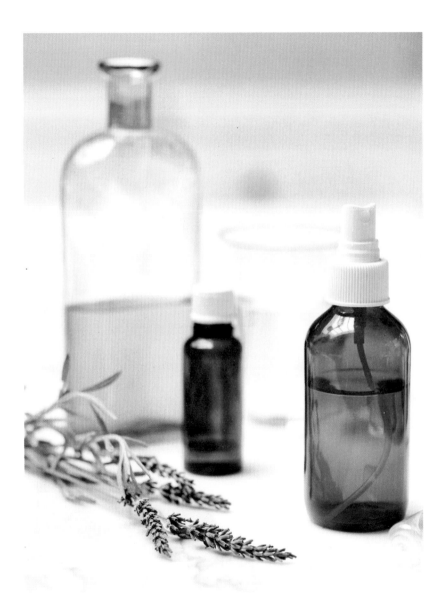

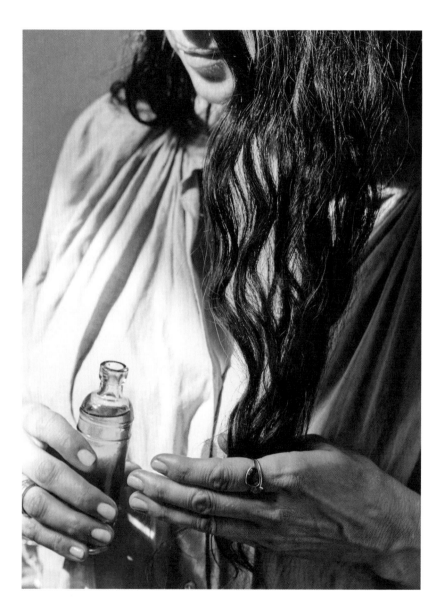

Powerful Locks Mask

As they age, many women experience a decrease in thyroid production. This affects the level of testosterone their bodies produce, which can in turn affect hair growth and thickness. This mask helps to stimulate hair growth and can also give your mane a boost if you have hair loss after pregnancy. In Ayurveda, bhringaraj, one of the main ingredients in this recipe, is known as the "king of hair" for how well it promotes hair growth, reduces balding, and stops premature graying.

For
Those with thinning hair

Recommended Use
Once or twice a month

2 to 3 teaspoons bhringaraj oil
2 to 3 ounces coconut or almond oil (depending on the length of your hair)

In a bowl, mix the bhringaraj oil and coconut or almond oil with enough warm water to form a thick paste. Cover your scalp with the paste, then massage the oil through your hair, from the scalp down to the ends. Leave on for 20 minutes, then lightly shampoo.

Silky Tresses Mask

Egg yolks are rich in fat and protein. They moisturize, fight frizz, and leave hair gleaming. You can put egg yolk directly on your hair for a quick shine boost, or make this simple mask with enzyme-rich honey to also help thicken your hair and leave it gorgeous and bouncy.

For

Dry, dull, or damaged hair. Also great to use if you regularly straighten or blow-dry your hair.

Recommended Use

Once a month

1 banana

1 egg yolk

2 tablespoons raw honey

1 tablespoon olive oil (optional; use only if you have dry hair)

Puree the banana in a blender (or give it a good mash with your hands), then transfer to a bowl. Fold in the egg yolk, honey, and olive oil (if using). Apply to your hair, starting at the scalp and working down to the ends. Leave on for 20 minutes, then wash out with your favorite shampoo. You may follow with conditioner if you like.

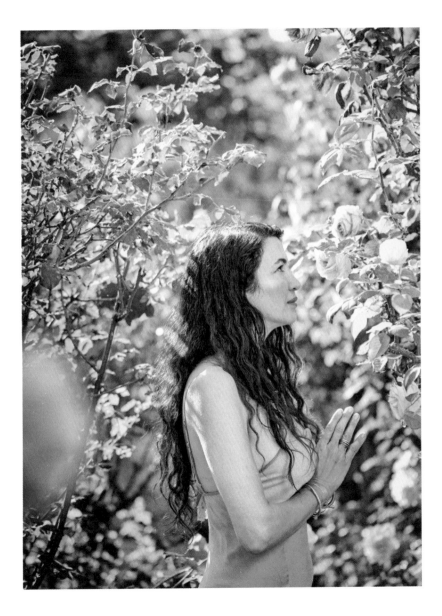

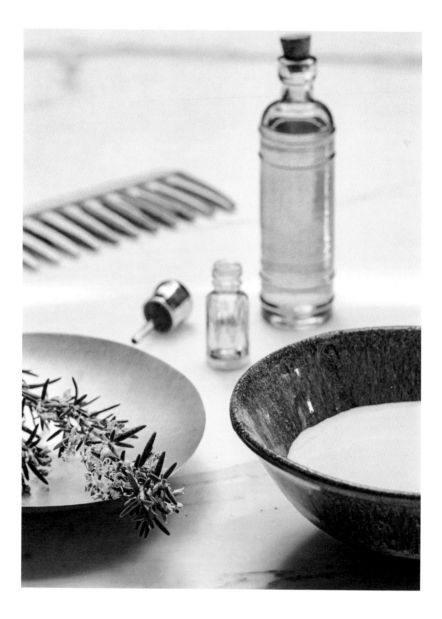

Simple Shampoo

Most traditional shampoos foam up because they are full of sulfates, which can irritate your skin (as you well know if you've ever gotten shampoo in your eyes!) and strip your hair of much-needed moisture. This nontoxic shampoo is easy to make. Store it in a glass jar and it will last for a couple of months. You'll also find that the healthier your hair becomes, the less often you'll need to shampoo.

For
All hair types

Recommended Use
As often as you typically shampoo

¼ cup coconut milk
¼ cup liquid castile soap (I like Dr. Bronner's)
20 drops of rosemary or peppermint essential oil
½ teaspoon olive or almond oil

Glass jar with stopper

Combine the coconut milk, soap, essential oil, and olive or almond oil in the glass jar. Shake well before each use, and shampoo as you normally would.

Gracious & Divine
Moisture Mask

Just as the earth dries out, we as women can also—stress and depleted diets can leave hair brittle so that it cracks and breaks instead of bending. This mask helps to replenish your hair with much-needed moisture so that it can be like the olive branch—supple and abundant. Olive oil is high in fat and oleic acid, which helps to nourish the strands of your hair from the inside out.

For

Dry to normal hair

Recommended Use

Once a month

½ avocado
3 tablespoons olive oil
½ cup plain yogurt

In a bowl, mash the avocado, then mix in the olive oil and yogurt, stirring until smooth and creamy. Apply to your hair, starting at the scalp and working down to the ends. Leave on for 20 minutes, then lightly shampoo.

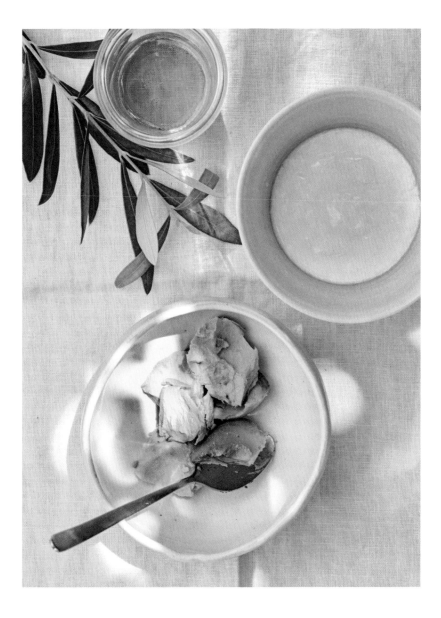

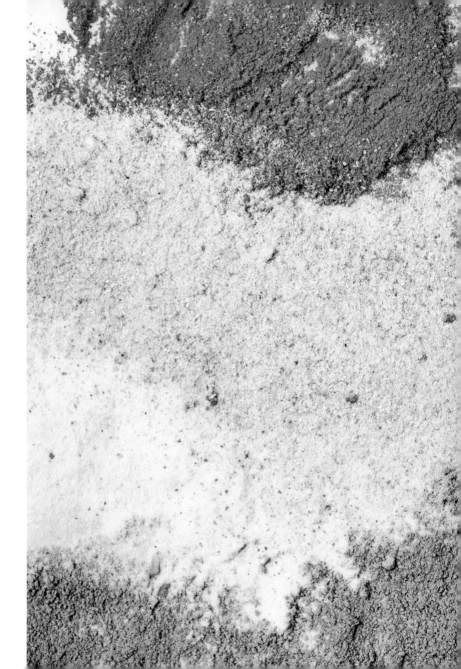

Face & Body Exfoliants

I first created my Sea Siren Scrub when camping with several women on Washington State's Orcas Island, a mystical place that inspired in me a gratitude for nature and all the wonderful women in my life. I mixed together coconut oil, shea butter, lemongrass, and a little bit of sugar, and we all spread it on our bodies and went into a sauna that had been built in the woods. I felt that we were connecting to the magical animals that give the island its name. We created a ritual around the moment, imagining ourselves as mermaids in tune with the whales. Whenever I use a scrub, I like to imagine that I am releasing what I don't need, taking off a layer of old living so that I can open myself up to letting in more sunshine and new light. Scrubbing away dead skin helps to remove toxins and release new energy.

In Iran, women used a *kiseh*, which is a loofah-like cloth, with *sefidab* ("white water"), a hardened chunk of minerals mixed with sheep fat, to keep their skin soft and glowing. Those can be hard to find in many parts of the world, but variations on Ayurvedic cleansing powders, called *ubtans*, are easy to make at home and provide the same benefits. Many store-bought exfoliants contain plastic microbeads, which do not decompose and remain in our rivers and oceans after they are washed down the drain. Chances are you already have many ingredients in your kitchen that can be used as natural exfoliants that won't harm your skin or the environment, such as those listed below.

Brown Rice

Brown rice is full of antioxidants, and it becomes a gentle exfoliant when you grind it uncooked in a coffee grinder until it has the consistency of coarse flour.

Cane Sugar

Sugar has smaller granules than salt, which means it is gentler on your skin than a salt scrub, and it is a natural source of glycolic acid, which helps remove dead skin cells.

Chickpea Flour

Chickpea flour absorbs extra oil, and is used in Ayurveda to lighten sun damage and even out overall skin tone.

Oat Flour

Oats have been used for centuries to calm skin irritations, and oat flour is an extremely gentle exfoliant for sensitive skin.

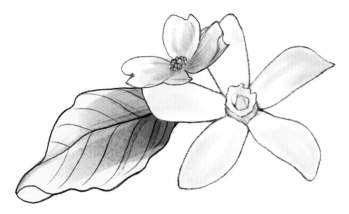

Blushing Bride
Chickpea Face Mask

Chickpea flour is wonderful in a mask, because it brightens, exfoliates, and draws out impurities from the skin. You can buy chickpea flour at a health food store, or make your own by grinding dried chickpeas in a coffee grinder until you get a fine, fairly uniform consistency. In this mask, the turmeric has melatonin-inhibiting enzymes that help lighten scars and discoloration. In India, brides use a chickpea mask as part of their wedding preparation ritual. Using this mask is a great way to pamper yourself before special occasions.

For
Normal to oily skin

Recommended Use
Once a week

5 tablespoons chickpea flour
1 tablespoon plain yogurt
¼ teaspoon turmeric
½ teaspoon sandalwood powder

In a bowl, mix the chickpea flour with enough water to form a paste. Then add the yogurt, turmeric, and sandalwood powder. Wet your face and apply the mask in a circular motion. Leave on for 15 minutes, then wash off with warm water.

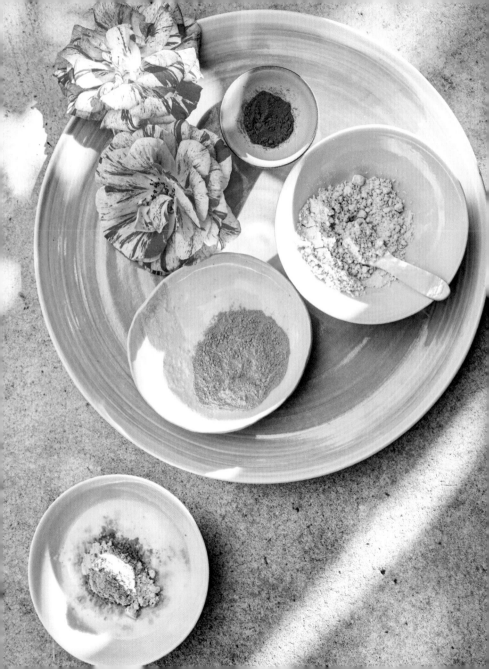

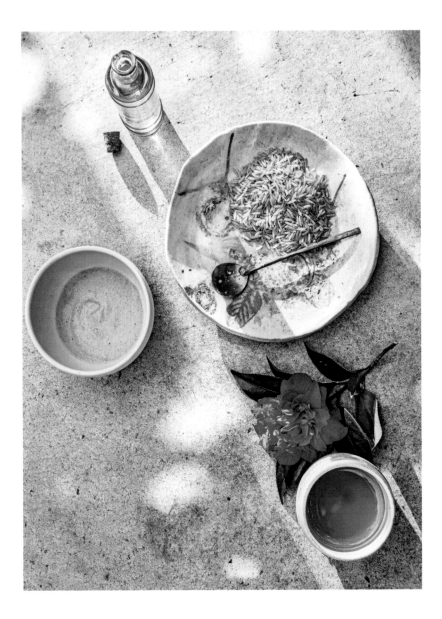

Heavenly Light Face Scrub

Sesame seeds are used often in Ayurvedic recipes for their high mineral content and conditioning aspects. Here, zinc-rich sesame oil is combined with brown rice to slough off dead skin cells; green tea provides a dose of anti-aging antioxidants. Use this scrub to remove the blockage of dull cells and reveal fresh new ones so that your skin casts a beautiful glow.

For
Normal to dry skin

Recommended Use
Once a month, or whenever you feel your skin needs exfoliation

2 tablespoons uncooked brown rice
Contents of 1 tea bag of green tea
1 tablespoon sesame seed oil

Grind the rice and tea to a fine powder in a coffee grinder and transfer to a bowl. Stir in the sesame oil. Wet your face and apply the scrub in a circular motion. Leave on for 20 minutes, then wash off with warm water.

Revitalizing Body Scrub

I like to think of this as a "Choose Your Own Adventure" treatment. The sugar-and-oil base makes a wonderful scrub on its own, but you can also modify it with additional ingredients to really target your skin type or just to make it more playful and delicious. Keeping a batch ready to go in a mason jar can add a little extra splendor to your shower on even the busiest days.

For

All skin types

Recommended Use

Once a week, or as needed

1 cup organic cane sugar
¼ cup coconut oil
¼ cup sunflower or almond oil
A few drops of vanilla essential oil
Modifications to your liking (optional; see opposite)

Mason jar with lid

Combine the sugar, coconut oil, sunflower or almond oil, essential oil, and your choice of modifications, if using, in the lidded mason jar and shake well to mix. Wet your skin and apply the scrub starting at the feet, always working upward and inward toward the heart. Concentrate on rough spots like knees and elbows. Rinse well, but to preserve the moisturizing properties, do not wash off with soap.

Modifications

- For a tropical scrub, add ½ papaya, pureed

- To target dry midwinter skin (and make your bathroom smell like the holidays), add 1 cup coffee grounds and 1 teaspoon cinnamon

- For extra brightening, add the juice of 1 lemon and 2 tablespoons raw honey

- To nourish sensitive skin, add 1 cup uncooked oats and 2 tablespoons raw honey

- To target feet and elbows, add the zest and juice of 1 lemon

- For extra moisturizing, add a mashed banana

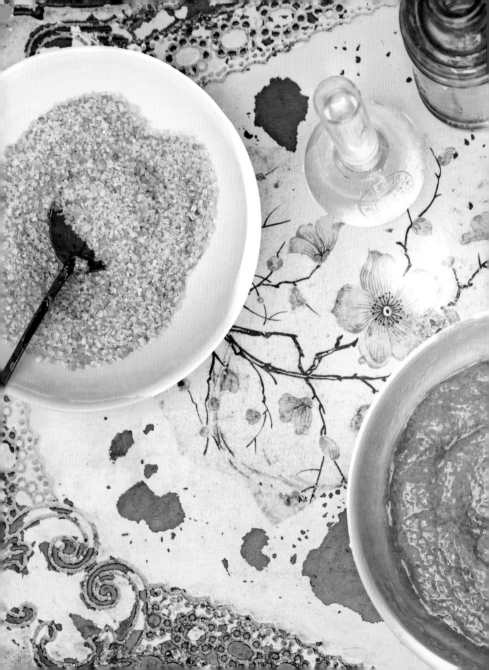

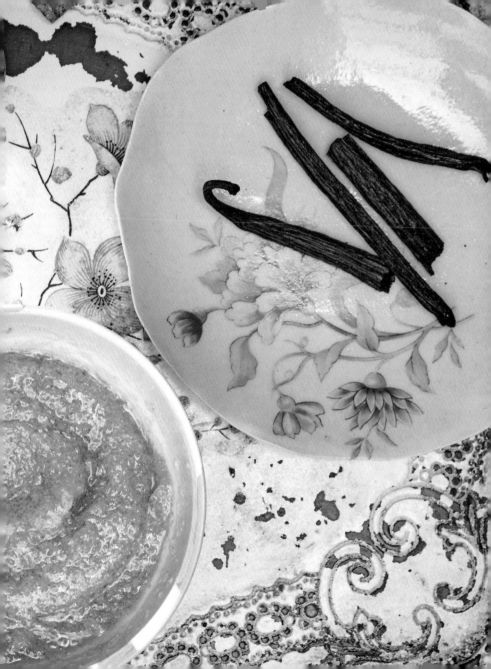

Balancing Bath

The five foods used in this pre-bath rub are
known for balancing the doshas (see page 51).

1 banana, mashed or pureed

1 teaspoon ghee (see Resources)

1 teaspoon plain yogurt

1 teaspoon raw honey

3 tablespoons milk, preferably raw (see page 21)

Fill the tub with water that is the ideal temperature
for you. Mix together the banana, ghee, yogurt,
honey, and milk and massage the rub into your skin
from your feet to your face. Then soak in the bath
for 20 minutes or more.

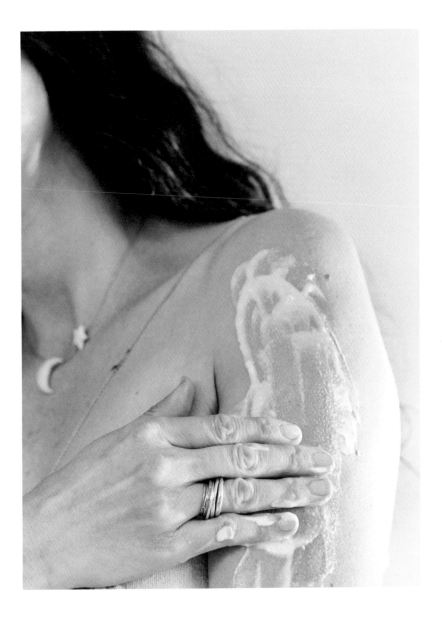

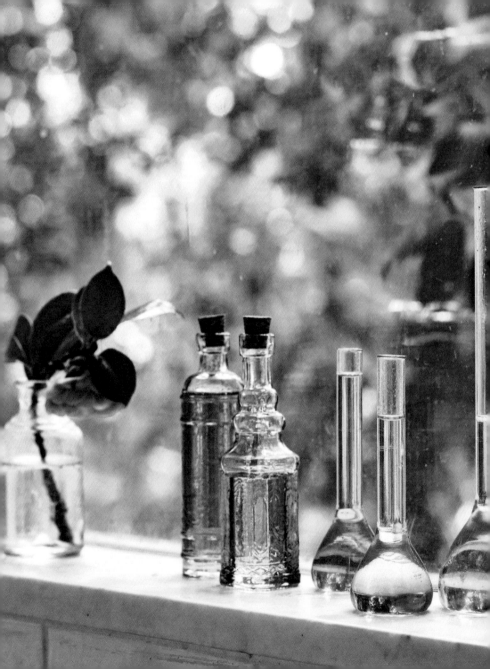

Oils for Hair, Face & Body

It might seem counterintuitive to put oil on your skin, but it's actually something your skin really needs. Just like shampoo strips the hair, most conventional cleansers strip the skin of its essential moisture. This affects the pH and microbiome of your skin, leaving it vulnerable to irritation and breakouts and speeding up the aging process. Because they are lipophilic—or fat loving—oils pass through the lipid layer of the skin faster than water-based moisturizers. The right oils will wake up your skin, soothe it, and help it glow.

Oil has devotional properties and has been used for centuries to anoint royalty. To use oils is to connect with the divine. Take a moment to savor the act of putting drops of it into your bath, the feeling of it being absorbed into your skin, of it being taken in through your hair and hands.

When using any oil, remember to take the time and intention to anoint yourself rather than just slather it on, so that you fully experience how luxurious oils can be. As with anything you are using on your skin or scalp for the first time, you may want to test for sensitivity by applying it to a small area of your inner arm, then waiting twenty-four hours to see if an irritation develops.

I like to have a variety of oils on hand to meet different skin and hair needs. All of these can be used alone or blended.

Almond Oil

Almond oil has been used by Ayurvedic practitioners for centuries. It is brimming with vitamin E, and massaging it on the skin below the eyes will help reduce dark circles.

Argan Oil

Argan oil is loaded with omega-6 fatty acids, linoleic acid, and vitamins A and E. It helps boost cell production and is anti-inflammatory, which is why it was historically used to treat bug bites and skin irritation.

Camellia Oil

Camellia oil is sometimes known as tea seed oil, because it comes from *Camellia sinensis*, the tea plant. It is mildly astringent, anti-inflammatory, and high in antioxidants, just like green tea.

Castor Oil

I use castor oil on my eyebrows and eyelashes, as it stimulates hair to grow back thicker and fuller. Using a clean mascara wand, I brush some on every night before bed. You can add it to your conditioner to help promote thicker hair.

Coconut Oil

Not only is coconut oil delicious, but it is also a rich, wonderful moisturizer for skin and hair, and it can be used to remove makeup. It is rich in fatty acids and lauric acid, which is antifungal and antibacterial. Coconut oil solidifies at room temperature, so when using it for masks, melt it in a small bowl set in warm water.

Jojoba Oil

Jojoba oil is wonderful as a base for face moisturizers. Native Americans use it to treat bruises and sores, and it is rich in iodine, which makes it antibacterial.

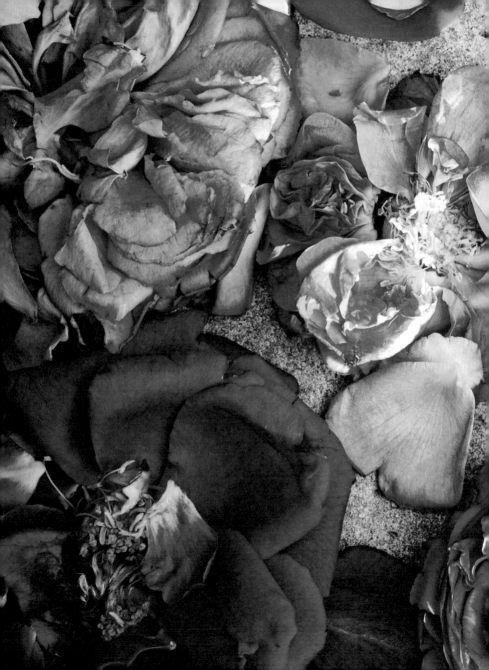

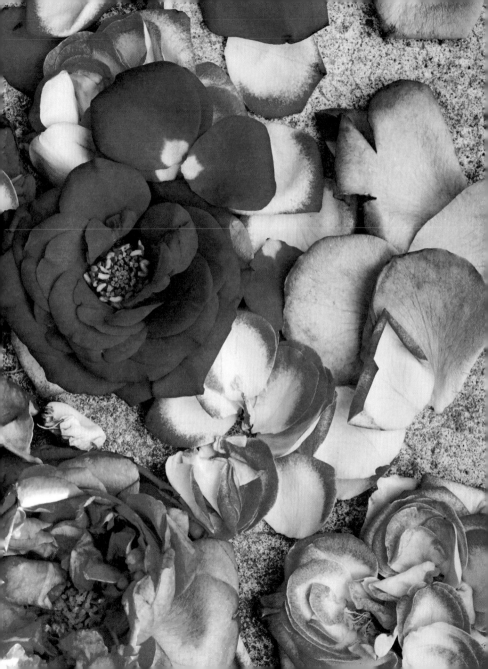

Kukui Nut Oil

A natural moisturizer that Hawaiian mermaids
have been using for centuries, kukui nut oil is a sun
worshipper's dream. It helps reduce sun damage
and also lightens stretch marks and treats scars.

Rose Hip Oil

Rose hip oil comes from wildflowers in the Himalayas
and is high in vitamins A and C. It is a powerful
anti-aging oil that was used by Greek goddesses
as part of their daily skin-care regimen.

Sea Buckthorn Oil

Sea buckthorn is a shrub that grows in Europe and
Asia and has long been used in Russia to help protect
skin against frigid winters. It heals wounds, reduces
inflammation, and helps build proteins in the skin.

Sesame Oil

Sesame oil has been used for thousands of years,
is mentioned in the Vedas, and is known as the
"queen of the oils." Sesame seeds are rich in
zinc, which is a potent antioxidant necessary for
producing collagen and retaining skin elasticity.

Shea Butter

A hydrating, rich, nourishing and grounding, skin-regenerating, tridosha moisturizer that helps to stimulate collagen production, shea butter will melt into an oil with the heat from your hands.

Sunflower Oil

Sunflower oil is a great base for body oils, and it is rich in vitamins A, D, and E.

Tamanu Oil

Tamanu trees are native to Southeast Asia, where people believed that the tree was a sacred gift of nature and that a god hid in its branches. Tamanu oil is anti-aging and can be used to treat age spots and stretch marks.

OILS FOR HAIR, FACE & BODY

Oil for Hair

Indian women traditionally condition their hair before washing it to protect it from the drying effects of shampoo, which makes complete sense. A lot of conventional shampoos can do more harm than good, with ingredients like sodium lauryl sulfates that strip the hair of its natural oils, which conventional conditioners do a poor job of replenishing. Oiling your hair is a simple practice that can help restore necessary moisture and bring lustrous shine back to your locks. It can be done weekly or monthly, as often as you need a deep conditioning, and you can continue to use your daily hair conditioner.

For

All hair types

Recommended Use

Once a week, or as often as you shampoo your hair

2 to 3 tablespoons coconut or sesame oil (depending on the length of your hair)

Brush or comb your hair thoroughly. Put the oil in a glass bowl. Heat a few inches of water in a saucepan and place the bowl in the water for a few minutes, or until the oil is warm. Starting with the crown of your head and working downward and outward, massage the oil into your scalp by pinching and releasing your

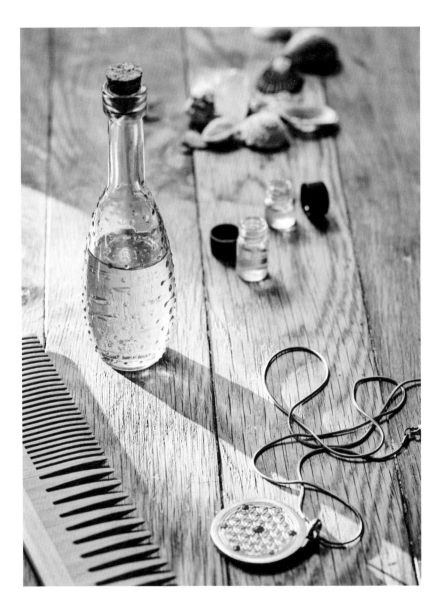

fingertips. Rub the oil through the strands of your hair, concentrating on the ends and adding more oil if needed. Leave on for 30 minutes, then wash your hair. For deep conditioning, you can leave the oil on overnight and wash it out in the morning.

To Combat Dandruff: Add a few drops of rose, lavender, geranium, or rosemary essential oil to your coconut or sesame oil, and really concentrate on spreading the oil on your scalp.

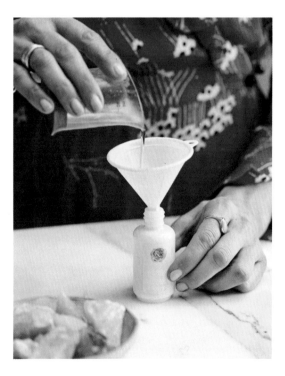

Nourishing Face Oil

Rose oil is nourishing, and it feeds and comforts the skin. It is inspired by the Hindu goddesses Lalita, the one who dwells in a forest of bliss and wanders free; Parvati, the daughter of a mountain who is moved by love; and Lakshmi, who offers the most lasting forms of wealth, integrity, empathy, compassion, and love. You can customize your face oil with your favorite essential oil.

For
Normal to dry skin

Recommended Use
Twice a day, or as needed

2 tablespoons jojoba oil
1 tablespoon kukui nut oil
1 tablespoon rose hip oil
1 tablespoon argan oil
1 teaspoon sea buckthorn oil
A few drops of vitamin E oil
A few drops of an essential oil that you like

4-ounce glass bottle with cap or stopper

Mix the oils and transfer to the glass bottle. Use a few drops to moisturize your skin in the morning, at night, or whenever it needs to be replenished.

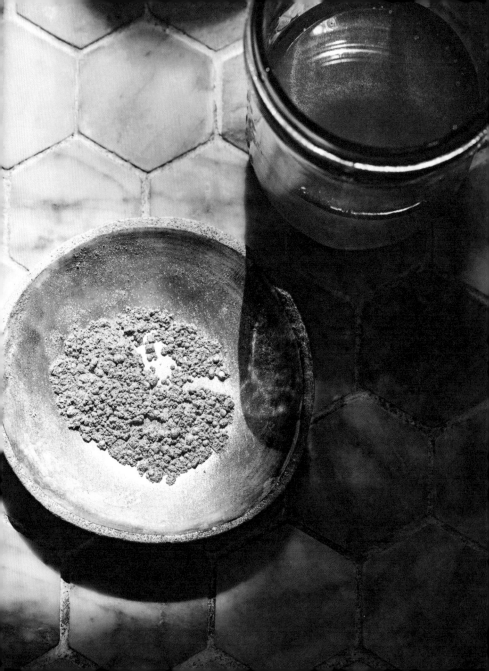

Shimmering Body Oil

This oil makes you absolutely glow! It's indulgent and fun, and it smells heavenly. Mica is a natural mineral dust that adds a hint of glimmer, making this body oil perfect for a date night or when you're wearing a beautiful dress and want to highlight your skin.

For
All skin types

Recommended Use
Use after bathing or before an evening out

2 teaspoons mica, either gold or bronze
1 tablespoon shea butter or coconut oil
3 ounces sunflower seed oil
5 drops of vanilla essential oil
   (or any essential oil you prefer)

4-ounce glass bottle with stopper

Using a funnel, pour the mica into the glass bottle. In a saucepan over low heat, melt the shea butter or coconut oil, then add it to the bottle. Pour in the sunflower seed oil and the vanilla essential oil, place the stopper in the bottle, and shake. Use your fingertips to apply lovingly to your shoulders, chest, and limbs.

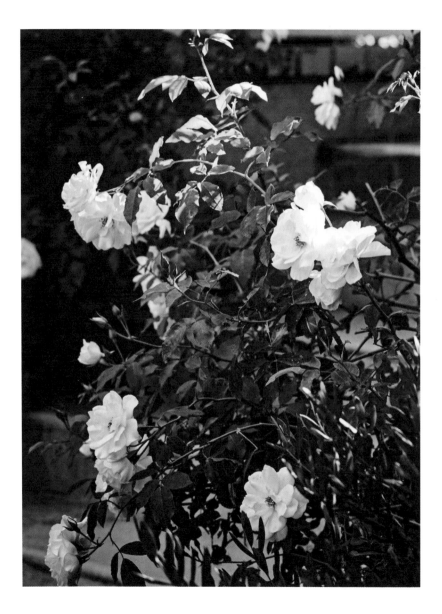

FURTHER READING

In addition to in my blog, *The Local Rose*, my writing has appeared on the following websites.

TheChalkboardMag.com
Goop.com
MindBodyGreen.com

These are a few books I recommend.

Ayurvedic Beauty Care: Ageless Techniques to Invoke Natural Beauty, by Melanie Sachs

The Complete Book of Essential Oils and Aromatherapy, by Valerie Ann Worwood

Natural Organic Hair and Skin Care, by Aubrey Hampton

RESOURCES

Learn more about holistic living and my products on TheLocalRose.com. In addition, these are the websites I frequently visit to shop for ingredients and seek out new insights and information.

Ayurveda
BanyanBotanicals.com
Chopra.com
SuryaSpa.com

To find an Ayurvedic practitioner in your area:
AyurvedaNAMA.org

Essential Oils
EdensGarden.com
LivingLibations.com

Ghee
AncientOrganics.com
FourthAndHeart.com

Herbs
BanyanBotanicals.com
DualSpices.com
MountainRoseHerbs.com
SusunWeed.com

Nontoxic Makeup
IliaBeauty.com
Kosas.com
RMSBeauty.com
VapourBeauty.com

Library of Congress Cataloging-in-Publication Data

Names: Rose, Shiva, author.
Title: Whole beauty : masks and scrubs : natural beauty recipes for
ultimate self-care / Shiva Rose.
Description: New York : Artisan, a division of
    Workman Publishing Co., Inc. [2019]
Identifiers: LCCN 2018030083 | ISBN 9781579659028
    (hardcover : alk. paper)
Subjects: LCSH: Essences and essential oils. | Beauty, Personal. |
    Face—Care and Hygiene. | Women—Health and hygiene.
Classification: LCC TP958 .R7753 2018 | DDC 661/.806—dc23
    LC record available at https://lccn.loc.gov/2018030083

Artisan books are available at special discounts when purchased in
bulk for premiums and sales promotions as well as for fund-raising or
educational use. Special editions or book excerpts also can be created
to specification. For details, contact the Special Sales Director at the
address below, or send an e-mail to specialmarkets@workman.com.

For speaking engagements, contact speakersbureau@workman.com.

Published by Artisan
A division of Workman Publishing Co., Inc.
225 Varick Street
New York, NY 10014-4381
artisanbooks.com

Artisan is a registered trademark of Workman Publishing Co., Inc.

This book has been adapted from *Whole Beauty* (Artisan, 2018).

Design adapted from CHD

Published simultaneously in Canada by Thomas Allen & Son, Limited

Printed in China
First printing, February 2019

10 9 8 7 6 5 4 3 2 1